STOMACH ULCER DIET

COOKBOOK

For Seniors

Leona Butler

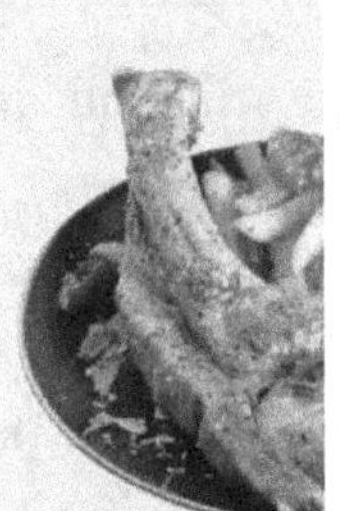

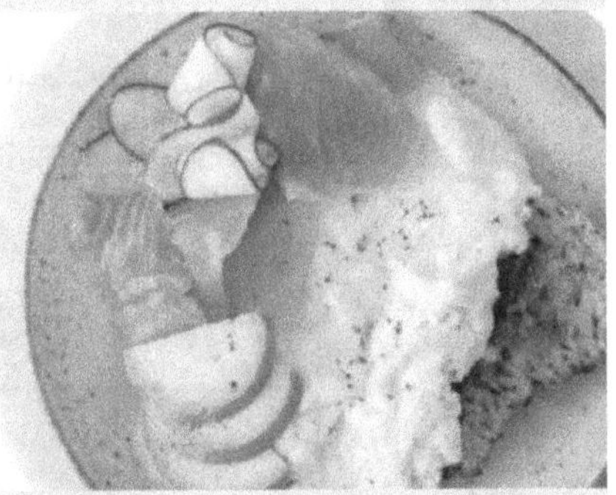

The Ultimate Recipes, Nutritional Guidance, And Easy To Digest Meals For Symptom Management And Inproved Quality Of Life

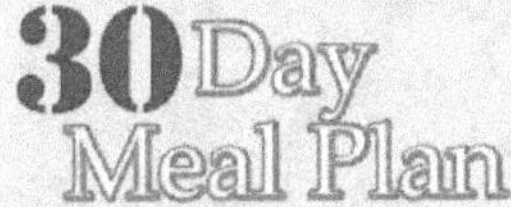

30 Day Meal Plan

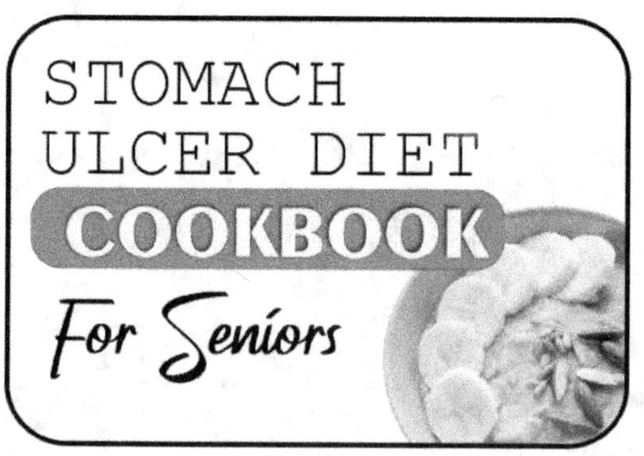
STOMACH
ULCER DIET
COOKBOOK
For Seniors

6 Easy Steps How To Use a Stomach Ulcer Diet Cookbook For Seniors

1. Research and Understand: Begin by researching foods that are beneficial and harmful for individuals with stomach ulcers. Understand which ingredients are soothing and which can aggravate the condition.

2. Consult Professionals: Talk to dietitians or healthcare providers who specialize in stomach ulcers to gather insights and recommendations for recipes.

3. Develop this Recipes: Create recipes that are gentle on the stomach, focusing on ingredients like lean proteins, whole grains, fruits, and vegetables. Avoid spicy, acidic, and fatty foods.

4. Include Variety: Ensure the cookbook includes a variety of recipes for different meals and occasions, including breakfast, lunch, dinner, and snacks. Incorporate different flavors and textures to keep meals interesting.

5. Provide Nutritional Information: Include nutritional information for each recipe, such as calorie count, macronutrient breakdown, and portion sizes, to help seniors make informed choices.

6. Consider Special Dietary Needs: Take into account any special dietary needs or restrictions that seniors may have, such as allergies or intolerances, and offer alternatives or substitutions where necessary.

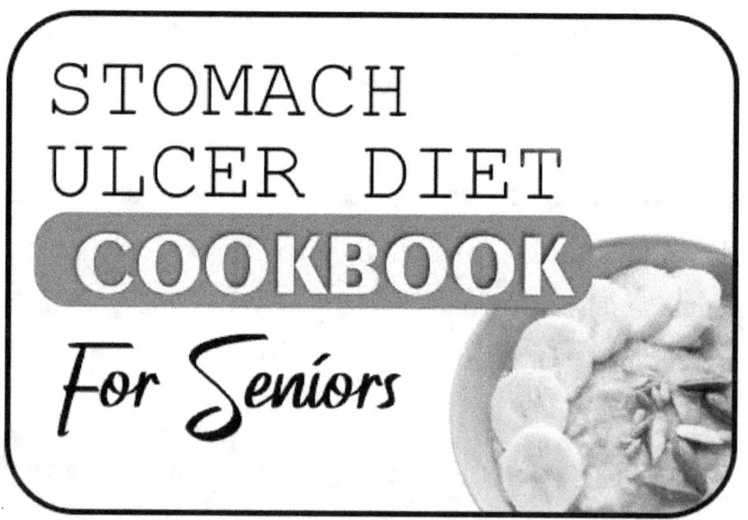

Table Of Content

Chapter 4: Lunch Recipes

1. GRILLED CHICKEN SALAD WITH BALSAMIC VINAIGRETTE:
2. LENTIL SOUP WITH CARROTS, CELERY, AND SPINACH:
3. TUNA SALAD WRAP WITH AVOCADO:
4. QUINOA SALAD WITH ROASTED VEGETABLES AND FETA CHEESE
5. TURKEY AND AVOCADO SANDWICH ON WHOLE GRAIN BREAD WITH A SIDE OF CARROT STICKS
6. CHICKPEA AND VEGETABLE STIR-FRY SERVED OVER BROWN RICE
7. SALMON SALAD WITH MIXED GREENS, STRAWBERRIES, AND LEMON VINAIGRETTE
8. VEGETABLE AND BEAN CHILI TOPPED WITH GREEK YOGURT AND CHOPPED CILANTRO:
9. WHOLE GRAIN PASTA WITH ROASTED CHERRY TOMATOES, GARLIC, AND BASIL
10. EGGPLANT AND HUMMUS WRAP WITH SPINACH, ROASTED RED PEPPERS, AND CUCUMBER SLICES

Chapter 5: Dinner Recipes

1. BAKED SALMON WITH STEAMED ASPARAGUS AND QUINOA
2. TURKEY MEATBALLS SERVED OVER WHOLE WHEAT SPAGHETTI WITH MARINARA SAUCE
3. STIR-FRIED TOFU WITH BROCCOLI, BELL PEPPERS, AND SNAP PEAS SERVED OVER BROWN RICE
4. GRILLED CHICKEN BREAST WITH ROASTED SWEET POTATOES AND SAUTÉED KALE
5. VEGGIE STIR-FRY WITH TOFU, BELL PEPPERS, ONIONS, AND SNOW PEAS OVER BROWN RICE
6. BAKED COD WITH ROASTED BRUSSELS SPROUTS AND WILD RICE PILAF
7. QUINOA STUFFED BELL PEPPERS WITH BLACK BEANS, CORN, AND SALSA
8. TURKEY AND VEGETABLE KEBABS SERVED WITH COUSCOUS
9. EGGPLANT PARMESAN WITH A SIDE OF MIXED GREEN SALAD
10. LENTIL AND VEGETABLE CURRY SERVED WITH WHOLE WHEAT NAAN BREAD

2024 EDITION

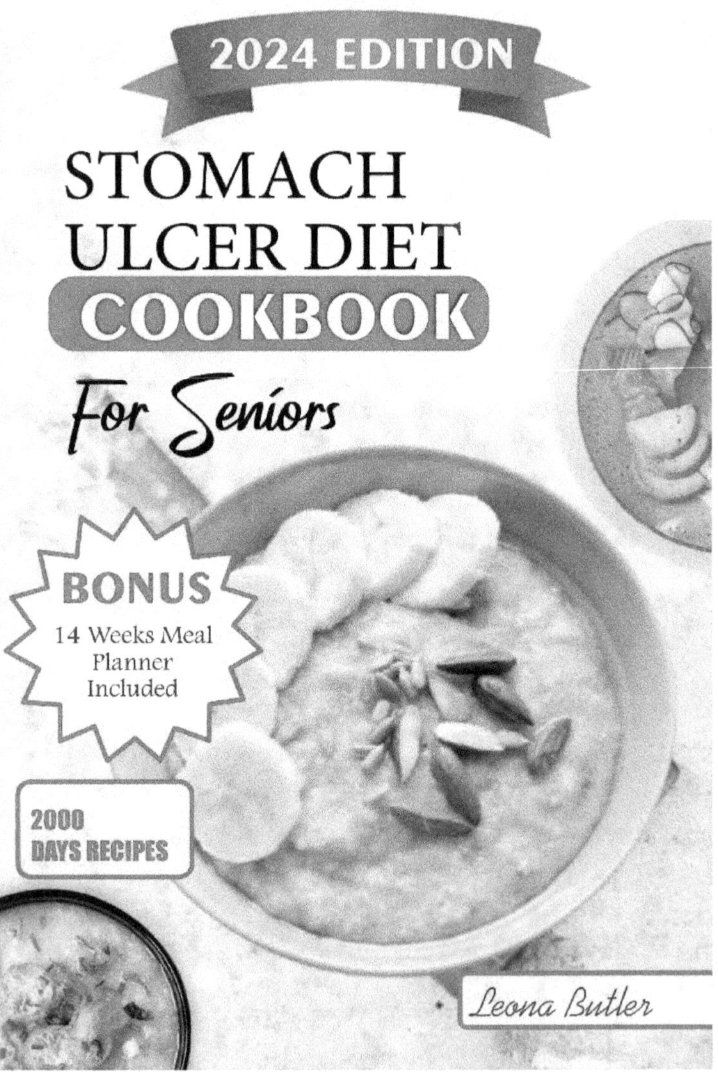
STOMACH ULCER DIET
COOKBOOK
For Seniors
BONUS
14 Weeks Meal
Planner
Included
2000
DAYS RECIPES
Leona Butler

Introduction

Introducing **Stomach Ulcers Cookbook for Seniors** a comprehensive culinary guide crafted to enhance the well-being of seniors navigating the challenges of stomach ulcers. This cookbook offers a treasure trove of benefits tailored to alleviate discomfort and promote healing. Inside, you'll discover a curated selection of gentle recipes meticulously designed to soothe sensitive stomachs while providing essential nutrients.

From easy-to-digest meals to nutritional guidance, each recipe is thoughtfully crafted to support seniors in managing their ulcer symptoms effectively. With a diverse array of flavorful dishes, this cookbook ensures that mealtimes remain enjoyable and varied, empowering seniors to maintain a balanced diet without sacrificing taste or satisfaction.

By embracing the recipes within these pages, seniors can find relief from discomfort, reduce the frequency of flare-ups, and ultimately enhance their quality of life. "Stomach

Ulcers Cookbook for Seniors" is more than just a cookbook; it's a companion on the journey to improved health and well-being.

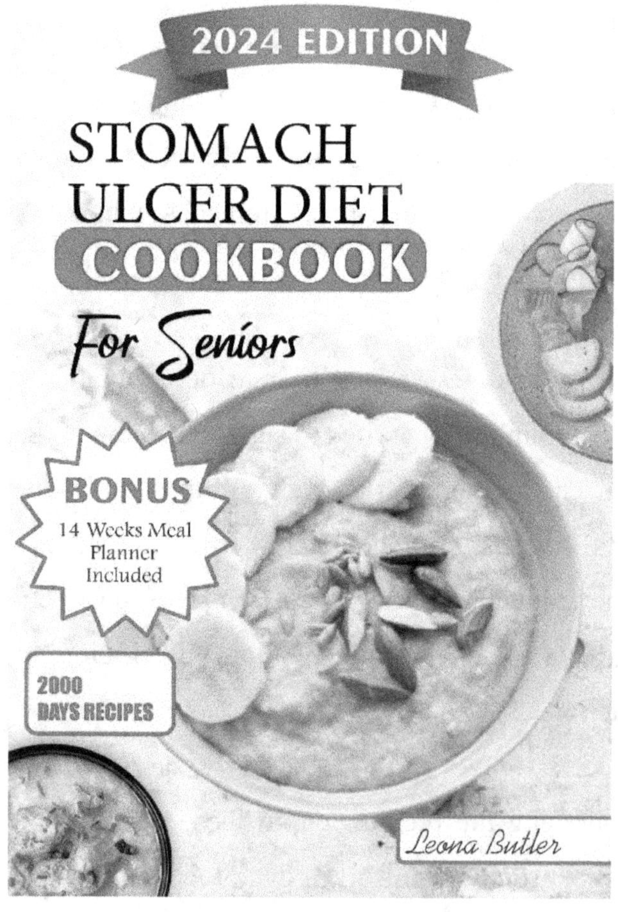

Chapter 1

What Are Stomach Ulcers?

Stomach ulcers, also known as peptic ulcers, are painful sores that develop on the lining of the stomach, small intestine, or esophagus. These ulcers can vary in size and severity, and they occur when the protective layer of mucus that lines the stomach and intestines becomes damaged or compromised, allowing stomach acid to erode the underlying tissue.

Types of Stomach Ulcers:

- Gastric Ulcers: These ulcers form in the lining of the stomach.
- Duodenal Ulcers: Found in the upper portion of the small intestine, duodenal ulcers are the most common type.

Stomach ulcers can manifest various symptoms, including:

1. Burning Pain: This pain typically occurs in the abdomen, often between meals and in the early hours of the morning.
2. Nausea and Vomiting: Some individuals may experience nausea and vomiting, particularly after eating.
3. Indigestion: Persistent indigestion or heartburn can be a sign of stomach ulcers.
4. Bloating: Bloating and feelings of fullness may occur, even after consuming small amounts of food.
5. Unintended Weight Loss: Severe ulcers can lead to weight loss due to a reduced appetite

Diagnosis often involves a combination of medical history review, physical examination, and diagnostic tests such as:

- Endoscopy: A thin, flexible tube with a camera is inserted into the digestive tract to visualize any ulcers directly.

- Barium X-ray: This imaging test involves swallowing a chalky liquid that coats the digestive tract, making ulcers visible on X-rays.

- Blood, Stool, or Breath Tests: These tests may be conducted to check for the presence of the bacterium Helicobacter pylori (H. pylori), a common cause of stomach ulcers.

Causes and Risk Factors:

Several factors can contribute to the development of stomach ulcers:

1. H. pylori Infection: This bacterium is a leading cause of stomach ulcers. It weakens the protective mucus layer, making the stomach more susceptible to damage from stomach acid.

2. Nonsteroidal Anti-inflammatory Drugs (NSAIDs): Regular use of medications like aspirin, ibuprofen, and naproxen can irritate the stomach lining, increasing the risk of ulcers.

3. Excessive Alcohol Consumption: Alcohol can irritate the stomach lining and increase acid production, contributing to ulcer formation.

4. Smoking: Smoking can weaken the stomach's protective lining, making it more susceptible to damage from acid.

5. Stress: While stress alone doesn't cause ulcers, it can exacerbate symptoms and delay healing.

6. Genetics: A family history of ulcers or a genetic predisposition to developing them can increase one's risk.

7. Age and Health Conditions: Older adults and those with certain health conditions such as liver, kidney, or lung disease may be more prone to developing stomach ulcers.

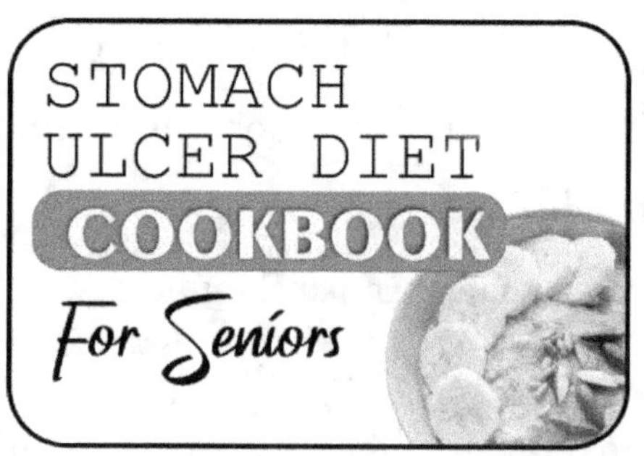

Chapter 2

The Role of Nutrition in Preventing Stomach Ulcers

Stomach ulcers, also known as peptic ulcers, are painful sores that develop on the lining of the stomach, small intestine, or esophagus. While factors like stress, smoking, and certain medications can contribute to their development, nutrition plays a crucial role in both prevention and management.

Importance of Diet in Stomach Ulcer Prevention

A well-balanced diet can help maintain the health of the digestive system and reduce the risk of stomach ulcers. Certain foods can either exacerbate ulcer symptoms or promote healing, making dietary choices essential in preventing and managing this condition.

1. Spicy Foods: Spices like chili powder, black pepper, and hot sauces can irritate the stomach lining, worsening ulcer symptoms.

2. Acidic Foods: Citrus fruits and juices, tomatoes, and vinegar can increase stomach acidity, potentially aggravating ulcers.

3. Highly Processed Foods: Processed foods like fast food, packaged snacks, and sugary treats often contain additives and preservatives that can irritate the stomach lining and delay ulcer healing.

4. Alcohol: Excessive alcohol consumption can erode the stomach lining and increase the risk of ulcers.

5. Caffeine: Coffee, tea, and caffeinated beverages stimulate acid production in the stomach, which may exacerbate ulcer symptoms.

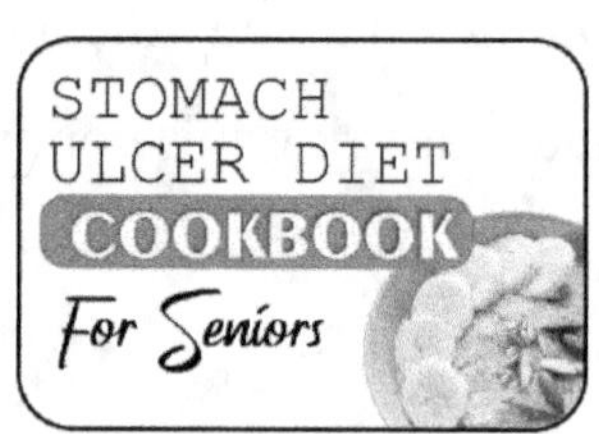

1. High-Fiber Foods: Fiber-rich foods like fruits, vegetables, whole grains, and legumes help regulate digestion and promote a healthy gut microbiome, which can aid in ulcer prevention and healing.

2. Probiotics: Yogurt, kefir, kimchi, and other fermented foods contain beneficial bacteria that support gut health and may help reduce the risk of ulcers.

3. Lean Proteins: Incorporating lean proteins such as poultry, fish, tofu, and beans into meals can provide essential nutrients without exacerbating ulcer symptoms.

4. Healthy Fats: Foods rich in omega-3 fatty acids, such as salmon, flaxseeds, and walnuts, have anti-inflammatory properties that may help soothe inflammation associated with ulcers.

5. Antioxidant-Rich Foods: Berries, leafy greens, nuts, and seeds are packed with antioxidants that can help protect the stomach lining from damage caused by oxidative stress.

Conclusion

In conclusion, while nutrition alone may not entirely prevent stomach ulcers, adopting a healthy diet can significantly reduce the risk of developing ulcers and alleviate symptoms in those already affected. Avoiding trigger foods like spicy and acidic items, alcohol, and caffeine, while incorporating fiber-rich foods, probiotics, lean proteins, healthy fats, and antioxidant-rich foods can support digestive health and contribute to ulcer prevention and management. Combined with other lifestyle modifications and medical treatment as needed, a balanced diet can play a vital role in promoting stomach health and overall well-being.

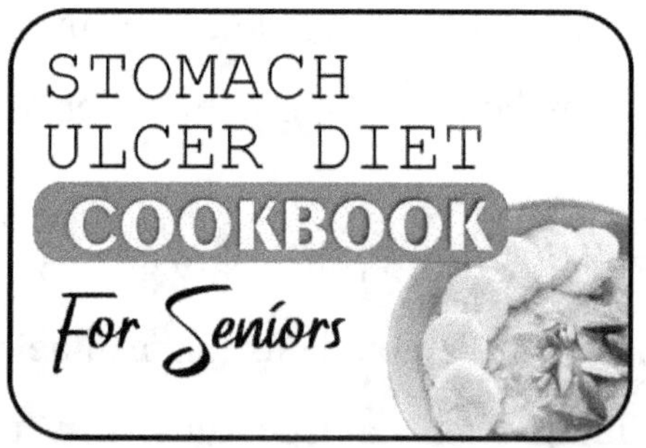

Chapter 3: Breakfast Recipes

1. Oatmeal with Sliced Bananas and Honey:

Ingredients:

- 1/2 cup rolled oats
- 1 cup water or milk
- 1 banana, sliced 1 tablespoon honey

Preparation:

1. In a small saucepan, heat the water or milk until it boils.
2. Stir in the rolled oats and decrease the heat to a simmer.
3. Cook for 5–7 minutes, stirring occasionally, until the oats are soft and creamy. Serve the oats in a bowl, topped with sliced bananas and drizzle with honey.

Nutritional Value:

- Oats: High in fiber, protein, and various nutrients such as manganese, phosphorus, magnesium, and zinc.

- Bananas: Rich in potassium, vitamin C, and vitamin B6.
- Honey: Contains antioxidants and may have antibacterial properties.

Cooking Time: 5-7 minutes

2. Whole Grain Toast with Almond Butter and Sliced Strawberries

Ingredients:

- 2 slices of whole grain bread
- 2 tablespoons almond butter 4-5 strawberries, sliced

Preparation:

1. Toast the whole-grain bread pieces till golden brown.
2. Spread 1 tablespoon almond butter onto each slice of toast. Place the sliced strawberries on top of the almond butter.

Nutritional Value:

- Whole grain bread: High in fiber, vitamins, and minerals.
- Almond butter: Rich in healthy fats, protein, fiber, vitamin E, magnesium, and calcium.
- Strawberries: Low in calories but high in vitamin C, manganese, folate, and antioxidants.

Cooking Time: 3-5 minutes (toasting time)

3. Scrambled Eggs with Spinach and Feta Cheese:

Ingredients:

- 2 eggs
- 1/2 cup fresh spinach, chopped
- 1/4 cup crumbled feta cheese Salt and pepper to taste

Preparation:

1. Crack the eggs into a bowl, season with salt and pepper, and whisk until thoroughly blended.

2. Heat a nonstick skillet over medium heat, then add the chopped spinach.

3. Cook the spinach for 1-2 minutes, until wilted.

4. Pour the whisked eggs into the skillet and gently scramble until thoroughly done. Sprinkle crumbled feta cheese over the scrambled eggs and serve hot.

Nutritional Value:

- Eggs: High in protein, vitamins, and minerals such as vitamin B12, riboflavin, and selenium.
- Spinach: Rich in iron, calcium, magnesium, and vitamins A, C, and K.
- Feta cheese: Contains calcium, phosphorus, and protein.

Cooking Time: 5-7 minutes

Enjoy your nutritious breakfast options!

4. Greek yogurt with sliced peaches and a drizzle of maple syrup

Ingredients:

- 1 cup Greek yogurt
- 1 ripe peach, sliced 1 tablespoon maple syrup

Preparation:

1. Wash the peach thoroughly and slice thinly.
2. Put 1 cup of Greek yogurt in a serving bowl.
3. Place the sliced peaches on top of the Greek yogurt.
4. Drizzle the maple syrup on the peaches and yogurt. Serve immediately and enjoy!

Nutritional Value:
- Greek yogurt (1 cup): Approximately 130 calories, 23g protein, 6g carbohydrates, 0g fat.
- Peach (1 medium): Approximately 60 calories, 1g protein, 15g carbohydrates, 0g fat.

- Maple syrup (1 tablespoon): Approximately 52 calories, 0g protein, 13g carbohydrates, 0g fat.

5. Buckwheat Pancakes:

Ingredients:

- 1 cup buckwheat flour
- 1 tablespoon baking powder
- 1/4 teaspoon salt
- 1 tablespoon honey or maple syrup
- 1 cup milk (dairy or plant-based) 1 large egg
- 1 tablespoon melted butter or oil
- Blueberries (as desired) Greek yogurt (as desired)

Preparation:

1. In a large mixing basin, combine buckwheat flour, baking powder, and salt.
2. In a separate bowl, whisk together the honey or maple syrup, milk, egg, and melted butter or oil. Pour the wet

ingredients into the dry ingredients and mix just until mixed. Don't overmix; a few lumps are fine.

3. Heat a nonstick skillet or griddle over medium heat and lightly coat with butter or oil.
4. Pour 1/4 cup batter into the skillet for each pancake.
5. Cook until bubbles appear on the surface of the pancake, then flip and cook until golden brown on the other side.
6. Serve the pancakes with blueberries and Greek yogurt.

Nutritional Value:

- Buckwheat is rich in fiber, protein, and various nutrients including manganese, magnesium, and iron.
- Blueberries are packed with antioxidants and vitamins C and K. Greek yogurt provides protein, calcium, and probiotics.

Cooking Time:
Approximately 20 minutes

6. Kale Pineapple Smoothie

Ingredients:

- 1 cup kale leaves, stems removed
- 1 cup fresh or frozen pineapple chunks
- 1 inch piece of ginger, peeled
- 1 cup coconut milk (or any milk of choice) Ice cubes (optional)

Preparation:

1. Combine all items in a blender.
2. Blend until smooth and creamy, adding more milk as needed to achieve the desired consistency. Taste and adjust the sweetness or flavor as needed by adding honey or additional pineapple.

Cooking Time:

Approximately 5 minutes

7. Cottage Cheese with Avocado and Cherry Tomatoes on Whole Grain Crackers

Ingredients:

- 1/2 cup cottage cheese
- 1 ripe avocado, sliced
- 1/2 cup cherry tomatoes, halved 4 whole grain crackers

Preparation:

1. Spread equal amounts of cottage cheese on each whole grain cracker.
2. Top each cracker with avocado slices and halved cherry tomatoes. Serve immediately.

Nutritional Value (per serving):
- Calories: Approximately 220
- Protein: 14g
- Carbohydrates: 18g
- Fat: 12g
- Fiber: 6g

Cooking Time: Preparation time: 5 minutes

8. Quinoa Breakfast Bowl with Apples, Cinnamon, and Nuts

Ingredients:

- 1/2 cup quinoa, rinsed
- 1 cup water
- apple, diced
- 1/2 teaspoon cinnamon
- tablespoons chopped nuts (such as almonds, walnuts, or pecans)

Preparation:

1. In a small saucepan, mix the quinoa and water. Bring to a boil, then reduce to a low heat and simmer for 15 minutes, or until the quinoa is cooked and the water has been absorbed.
2. Fluff cooked quinoa with a fork before transferring to a bowl.
3. Top with diced apples, cinnamon, and chopped nuts. Mix thoroughly and serve warm.

Nutritional Value (per serving):

- Calories: Approximately 350

- Protein: 9g

- Carbohydrates: 55g

- Fat: 11g

- Fiber: 7g

Cooking Time:

Preparation time: 5 minutes

Cooking time: 15 minutes

9. Poached Eggs over Whole Grain English Muffins with Sautéed Spinach and Mushrooms

Ingredients:

- 2 whole grain English muffins

- 4 large eggs

- 2 cups fresh spinach leaves

- 1 cup sliced mushrooms

- 1 tablespoon olive oil Salt and pepper to taste

Preparation:

1. Divide the English muffins in half and toast lightly.

2. In a skillet, heat the olive oil over medium heat. Sauté the sliced mushrooms until cooked, about 5 minutes.

3. Cook until the spinach is wilted, which should take around 2 minutes. Season with salt and pepper to taste.

4. Poach the eggs while the vegetables cook by bringing a pot of water to a low simmer. Crack an egg into a small bowl or ramekin. Carefully place each egg in the simmering water, cooking for 3-4 minutes for a runny yolk or longer for a firmer yolk.

5. Place the toasted English muffin halves on a platter. Top each half with sautéed spinach and mushrooms.

6. Use a slotted spoon to remove the poached eggs from the water and drain any excess water.

7. Put one poached egg on each English muffin half.

8. Season with more salt and pepper if required. Serve immediately.

Cooking Time: Approximately 15 minutes.

10. Chia Seed Pudding with Mixed Berries and a Dollop of Greek Yogurt

Ingredients:

- 1/4 cup chia seeds
- 1 cup unsweetened almond milk (or any milk of your choice)
- 1 tablespoon maple syrup or honey (optional, for sweetness)
- 1/2 teaspoon vanilla extract
- 1 cup mixed berries (such as strawberries, blueberries, raspberries)
- 1/4 cup Greek yogurt

Preparation:

1. In a mixing dish, add the chia seeds, almond milk, maple syrup (if using), and vanilla extract. Stir thoroughly to mix. Allow the mixture to sit for 5 minutes before stirring again to avoid clumping. Cover the bowl and chill for at least 2 hours, preferably overnight, to allow

the chia seeds to absorb the liquid and thicken into a pudding-like texture.

2. Before serving, whisk the chia seed pudding to ensure that it is properly combined and creamy.
3. Divide the pudding amongst serving bowls or glasses.
4. Garnish each bowl with mixed berries and a dollop of Greek yogurt. Serve cold.

Nutritional Value: Chia seeds are rich in fiber, omega-3 fatty acids, and various micronutrients. Berries are packed with antioxidants, vitamins, and fiber, while Greek yogurt adds protein and probiotics to the dish. This pudding is a nutritious and delicious breakfast or snack option.

Cooking Time: Approximately 2 hours for chilling, but active preparation time is minimal.

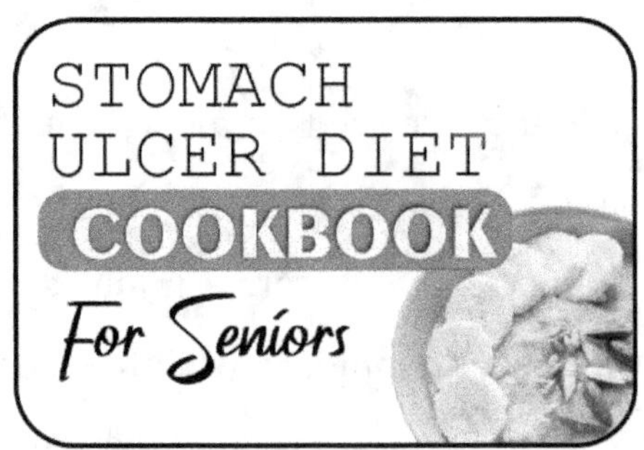

Chapter 4: Lunch Recipes

1. Grilled Chicken Salad with Balsamic Vinaigrette:

Ingredients:

- 200g grilled chicken breast
- 4 cups mixed greens
- 1 cup cherry tomatoes, halved
- cucumber, sliced
- tablespoons balsamic vinaigrette Salt and pepper to taste

Preparation:

1. Season the chicken breasts with salt and pepper.
2. Grill the chicken breasts for 6-8 minutes per side, or until cooked through.
3. In a large mixing bowl, combine mixed greens, cherry tomatoes, and cucumber slices.
4. Slice the grilled chicken breast and mix it into the salad.

5. Drizzle with balsamic vinaigrette and toss to coat. Serve immediately.

Nutritional Value:

- Calories: 350

- Protein: 35g

- Carbohydrates: 15g

- Fat: 15g

- Fiber: 5g

Cooking Time:

15-20 minutes

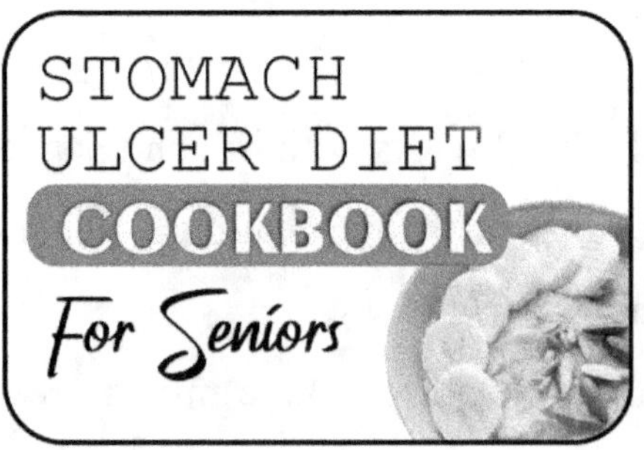

2. Lentil Soup with Carrots, Celery, and Spinach:

Ingredients:

- cup dried lentils
- carrots, diced
- 2 celery stalks, diced
- 2 cups spinach leaves
- 4 cups vegetable broth Salt and pepper to taste

Preparation:

1. Rinse the lentils with cool water.
2. In a large pot, mix lentils, carrots, celery, and vegetable broth.
3. Bring to a boil, then reduce the heat and simmer for 20-25 minutes, or until the lentils are cooked.
4. Stir in the spinach leaves and simmer for another 5 minutes, or until wilted.
5. Season with salt and pepper to taste. Serve hot.

Nutritional Value:

- Calories: 250
- Protein: 18g
- Carbohydrates: 45g
- Fat: 1g
- Fiber: 15g

Cooking Time:

30-35 minutes

3. Tuna Salad Wrap with Avocado:

Ingredients:

- 1 can (5 oz) tuna, drained
- 1 whole wheat tortilla
- 1/2 avocado, sliced
- 1 cup lettuce
- Salt and pepper to taste

Preparation:

1. In a bowl, combine the drained tuna, salt, and pepper.
2. Place a whole wheat tortilla on a flat surface.
3. Spread the tuna mixture evenly across the tortilla.
4. Top with lettuce and sliced avocado.
5. Roll the tortilla tightly into a wrap.
6. If desired, cut the wrap in half diagonally.

Nutritional Value:

- Calories: 300
- Protein: 25g
- Carbohydrates: 25g
- Fat: 12g
- Fiber: 8g

4. Quinoa Salad with Roasted Vegetables and Feta Cheese

Ingredients:

- cup quinoa
- cups mixed vegetables (such as bell peppers, zucchini, and cherry tomatoes), diced
- 2 tablespoons olive oil
- Salt and pepper to taste
- 1/2 cup feta cheese, crumbled
- Fresh herbs (such as parsley or basil), chopped

Preparation:

1. Preheat the oven to 400 °F (200 °C).
2. Rinse the quinoa with cold water and cook according to the package directions.
3. In a large bowl, combine the diced veggies, olive oil, salt, and pepper.

4. Place the vegetables on a baking sheet and roast in the preheated oven for 20-25 minutes, or until soft and slightly browned.

5. After the quinoa and vegetables have cooked, put them in a big serving bowl.

6. Toss in the crumbled feta cheese and chopped fresh herbs until well combined. Serve the quinoa salad warm or room temperature.

Nutritional Value:

- Quinoa is a good source of protein and fiber.
- Vegetables provide essential vitamins and minerals.
- Feta cheese adds protein and calcium to the dish.

Cooking Time: Approximately 30-35 minutes.

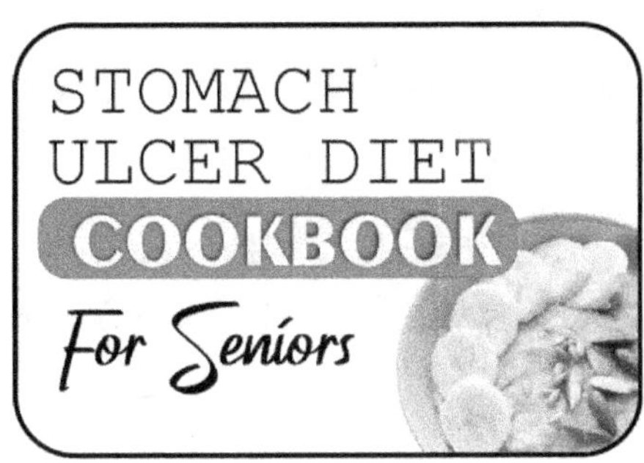

5. Turkey and Avocado Sandwich on Whole Grain Bread with a Side of Carrot Sticks

Ingredients:

- 4 slices whole grain bread
- 8 slices roasted turkey breast
- 1 avocado, sliced
- 1 cup carrot sticks
- Mustard or mayonnaise (optional)

Preparation:

1. Toast the whole grain bread pieces as desired.
2. Spread mustard or mayonnaise on one side of each slice of bread, if desired.
3. Layer the roasted turkey breast and avocado slices on two slices of toast.
4. Cover each sandwich with the remaining bread slices. Serve the sandwiches with a side of carrot sticks.

Nutritional Value:

- Whole grain bread provides fiber and complex carbohydrates.
- Turkey is a lean source of protein.
- Avocado offers healthy fats and vitamins.
- Carrot sticks are rich in beta-carotene and fiber.

Cooking Time: Approximately 10 minutes.

6. Chickpea and Vegetable Stir-Fry served over Brown Rice

Ingredients:

- 1 cup brown rice
- can (15 oz) chickpeas, drained and rinsed
- cups mixed vegetables (such as bell peppers, broccoli, and snap peas), chopped
- 2 tablespoons soy sauce
- 1 tablespoon sesame oil
- tablespoon olive oil
- cloves garlic, minced

- 1 teaspoon ginger, grated
- Salt and pepper to taste
- Sesame seeds for garnish (optional) Green onions, chopped for garnish (optional)

Preparation:

1. Cook brown rice according to the package instructions.
2. In a large skillet or wok, heat the olive oil over medium heat. Sauté minced garlic and grated ginger for 1-2 minutes, until fragrant.
3. Stir-fry the mixed vegetables in the skillet for 5-6 minutes, or until soft and crisp.
4. Stir in the drained chickpeas and simmer for an additional 2-3 minutes.
5. In a small bowl, combine soy sauce and sesame oil. Pour the sauce over the vegetables and chickpeas, tossing to cover.
6. Season with salt and pepper to taste.
7. Serve the stir-fry over cooked brown rice, topped with sesame seeds and chopped green onions if preferred.

Nutritional Value:

- Brown rice provides fiber and complex carbohydrates.

- Chickpeas are high in protein and fiber.

- Vegetables offer vitamins, minerals, and fiber.

- Sesame oil adds flavor and healthy fats.

Cooking Time: Approximately 25-30 minutes.

7. Salmon Salad with Mixed Greens, Strawberries, and Lemon Vinaigrette

Ingredients:

- 2 salmon fillets (6 oz each)
- 4 cups mixed greens
- cup strawberries, sliced
- tablespoons olive oil
- 1 tablespoon lemon juice
- 1 teaspoon Dijon mustard Salt and pepper to taste

Preparation:

1. Preheat the oven to 400°F (200°C).
2. Season salmon fillets with salt and pepper.
3. Arrange the salmon fillets on a baking pan lined with parchment paper.
4. Bake for 12-15 minutes, until thoroughly cooked.
5. In a small mixing bowl, combine olive oil, lemon juice, Dijon mustard, salt, and pepper to make the vinaigrette.
6. In a large salad dish, combine the mixed greens and sliced strawberries with the vinaigrette. Divide the salad amongst plates and top with a baked salmon fillet. Serve immediately.
7. Nutritional Value:
8. Salmon is a great source of protein, omega-3 fatty acids, and vitamins.
9. Mixed greens and strawberries provide fiber, vitamins, and antioxidants.
10. Olive oil adds healthy fats to the dish.

Cooking Time:
Approximately 20 minutes

Ingredients:

- 1 tablespoon olive oil
- onion, diced
- cloves garlic, minced
- bell pepper, diced
- carrots, diced
- 1 zucchini, diced
- 1 can (15 oz) diced tomatoes
- 1 can (15 oz) black beans, drained and rinsed
- can (15 oz) kidney beans, drained and rinsed
- cups vegetable broth
- 1 tablespoon chili powder
- 1 teaspoon cumin
- Salt and pepper to taste
- Greek yogurt and chopped cilantro for topping

Preparation:

1. In a large pot, heat the olive oil over medium heat.
2. Sauté diced onion and minced garlic until softened, about 5 minutes.
3. Cook for a further 5 minutes after adding the diced bell pepper, carrots, and zucchini.
4. Mix in the diced tomatoes, black beans, kidney beans, vegetable broth, chili powder, cumin, salt, and pepper.
5. Bring the chili to a simmer and cook for about 20-25 minutes, stirring occasionally.
6. Taste and adjust the seasoning as needed.
7. Serve the chili hot, with a dollop of Greek yogurt and chopped cilantro.

Nutritional Value:

This chili is packed with fiber, protein, vitamins, and minerals from the beans and vegetables. Greek yogurt adds protein and calcium, while cilantro provides additional flavor and some antioxidants.

Cooking Time:

Approximately 40 minutes

9. Whole Grain Pasta with Roasted Cherry Tomatoes, Garlic, and Basil

Ingredients:

- 200g whole grain pasta
- 250g cherry tomatoes
- 3 cloves garlic, minced
- 1/4 cup fresh basil leaves, chopped
- 2 tablespoons olive oil Salt and pepper to taste

Preparation:

1. Preheat the oven to 200 °C (400°F).
2. On a baking sheet, toss the cherry tomatoes with 1 tablespoon olive oil, minced garlic, salt and pepper.
3. Roast the tomatoes in a warm oven for 20-25 minutes, or until tender and slightly caramelized.
4. Cook whole grain pasta according to package directions until al dente.

5. Drain the pasta and combine it with the roasted cherry tomatoes, chopped basil leaves, and the remaining olive oil.

6. Serve hot, garnished with more basil leaves if desired.

Nutritional Value:

- Calories: Approximately 400 per serving

- Protein: Approximately 10g per serving

- Carbohydrates: Approximately 60g per serving

- Fat: Approximately 15g per serving Fiber: Approximately 10g per serving

Cooking Time:

Approximately 25-30 minutes

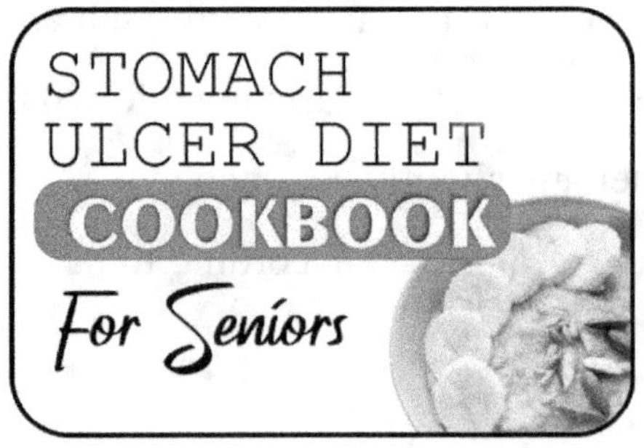

10. Eggplant and Hummus Wrap with Spinach, Roasted Red Peppers, and Cucumber Slices

Ingredients:

- 1 large eggplant, sliced into rounds
- 4 whole wheat wraps or tortillas
- cup hummus
- cups fresh spinach leaves
- 1 cup roasted red peppers, sliced 1 cucumber, thinly sliced

Preparation:

1. Preheat a grill or grill pan over medium-high heat.
2. Brush the eggplant slices with olive oil and season with salt and pepper.
3. Grill the eggplant slices for 4-5 minutes per side, or until they are soft and have grill marks.
4. Warm up the whole wheat wraps or tortillas in a dry skillet or microwave for a few seconds.
5. Spread 1/4 cup of hummus on each wrap.

6. Add grilled eggplant pieces, fresh spinach leaves, roasted red pepper slices, and cucumber slices.

7. Roll the wraps firmly, folding in the sides as you go. Slice in half diagonally and serve.

Nutritional Value:

- Calories: Approximately 350 per wrap

- Protein: Approximately 10g per wrap

- Carbohydrates: Approximately 45g per wrap

- Fat: Approximately 15g per wrap Fiber: Approximately 10g per wrap

Cooking Time:

Approximately 20-25 minutes (including grilling time for the eggplant)

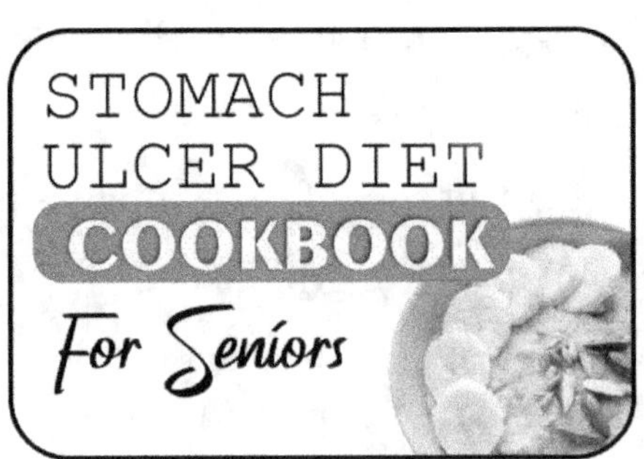

Chapter 6: Dinner Recipes

1. Baked Salmon with Steamed Asparagus and Quinoa

Ingredients:

- 2 salmon fillets (about 6 oz each)
- 1 bunch of asparagus (about 1 lb)
- 1 cup quinoa
- Salt and pepper to taste
- Olive oil
- Lemon wedges for serving

Preparation:

1. Preheat the oven to 400°F (200°C).
2. Rinse the quinoa in cold water and drain thoroughly. In a saucepan, add 2 cups water, quinoa, and a touch of salt. Bring to a boil, then reduce to a low heat, cover, and

simmer for 15 minutes, or until the quinoa is cooked and the water has been absorbed.

3. While the quinoa cooks, prepare the fish. Arrange the salmon fillets on a baking pan lined with parchment paper. Drizzle with olive oil, then season with salt and pepper.

4. Trim the woody ends of the asparagus spears. Arrange the asparagus on another baking sheet, drizzle with olive oil, and season with salt and pepper.

5. Place both baking sheets in the oven and bake for 12-15 minutes, or until the salmon is done and the asparagus is tender.

6. Serve the baked salmon and asparagus over cooked quinoa, topped with lemon wedges.

Nutritional Value:

- Salmon: Rich in omega-3 fatty acids, protein, and vitamin D.

- Asparagus: High in fiber, folate, and vitamins A, C, and K.

- Quinoa: High in protein, fiber, and various vitamins and minerals.

Ingredients:

- 1 lb ground turkey
- 1/2 cup breadcrumbs
- 1/4 cup grated Parmesan cheese
- egg
- cloves garlic, minced
- 1 teaspoon dried oregano
- 1 teaspoon dried basil
- Salt and pepper to taste
- 8 oz whole wheat spaghetti
- 2 cups marinara sauce Fresh basil leaves for garnish

Preparation:

1. Preheat the oven to 400°F (200°C).
2. In a large mixing bowl, combine ground turkey, breadcrumbs, Parmesan cheese, egg, chopped garlic,

dried oregano, dried basil, salt, and pepper. Mix until thoroughly mixed.

3. Roll the mixture into 1-2 tablespoon-sized meatballs and place on a parchment-lined baking sheet.

4. Bake the meatballs in the preheated oven for 20-25 minutes, or until well cooked and browned.

5. While the meatballs bake, prepare the whole wheat spaghetti according to package directions.

6. In a saucepan, cook the marinara sauce over medium heat.

7. Once the meatballs are cooked, combine them with the marinara sauce and simmer for a few minutes.

8. Serve the turkey meatballs and marinara sauce over cooked whole wheat spaghetti, topped with fresh basil.

Cooking Time:

Approximately 45 minutes

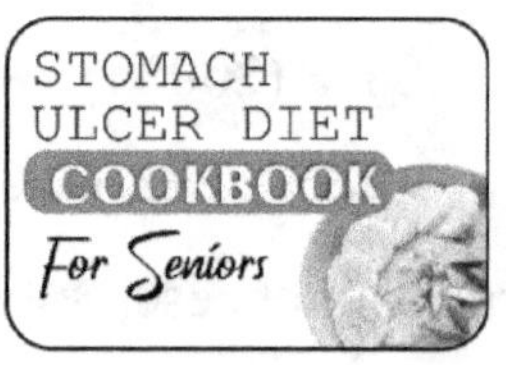

Ingredients:

- 200g firm tofu, drained and cubed
- cup broccoli florets
- 1/2 red bell pepper, thinly sliced
- 1/2 yellow bell pepper, thinly sliced
- 1/2 cup snap peas
- cups cooked brown rice
- 2 cloves garlic, minced
- 2 tablespoons soy sauce (low sodium recommended)
- 1 tablespoon sesame oil
- 1 tablespoon vegetable oil
- 1 teaspoon ginger, minced Salt and pepper to taste

Cooking Time:

Approximately 20 minutes

Preparation:

1. In a large skillet or wok, heat the vegetable oil over medium-high.
2. Cook tofu cubes till golden brown on all sides, about 5-7 minutes. Remove the tofu from the skillet and put aside.
3. In the same skillet, heat the sesame oil and sauté the garlic and ginger until fragrant, about 1 minute.
4. Add the bell peppers, broccoli, and snap peas to the skillet. Stir-fry for 3-4 minutes, until the vegetables are soft and crisp.
5. Return the tofu to the skillet and add the soy sauce. Stir well to incorporate, then simmer for another 2 minutes.
6. Serve the stir-fried tofu and vegetables with cooked brown rice. Season with salt and pepper to taste.

Nutritional Value:
- Calories: Approximately 350 per serving
- Protein: Approximately 15g
- Carbohydrates: Approximately 40g
- Fat: Approximately 15g

4. Grilled Chicken Breast with Roasted Sweet Potatoes and Sautéed Kale

Ingredients:

- 2 chicken breasts (about 200g each), boneless and skinless
- 2 medium sweet potatoes, peeled and diced
- 4 cups kale, stems removed and chopped
- 2 tablespoons olive oil
- 1 teaspoon paprika
- 1/2 teaspoon garlic powder Salt and pepper to taste

Preparation:

1. Preheat the grill to medium-high heat.
2. Season the chicken breasts with paprika, garlic powder, salt, and pepper.
3. Grill chicken breasts for 6-8 minutes on each side, or until internal temperature reaches 165°F (75°C). Remove from the grill and allow it rest for 5 minutes before slicing.

4. Meanwhile, preheat the oven to 400°F (200° C).

5. Toss the chopped sweet potatoes with olive oil, salt, and pepper. Place them in a single layer on a baking sheet and roast for 20-25 minutes, or until soft and slightly crusty.

6. In a separate skillet, warm the olive oil over medium heat. Sauté the kale until wilted, about 5-7 minutes.

7. Serve grilled chicken with roasted sweet potatoes and sautéed greens.

Nutritional Value:

- Calories: Approximately 400 per serving
- Protein: Approximately 30g
- Carbohydrates: Approximately 30g
- Fat: Approximately 15g

Cooking Time:

Approximately 40 minutes

Ingredients:

- 200g firm tofu, drained and cubed
- 1/2 red bell pepper, thinly sliced
- 1/2 green bell pepper, thinly sliced
- 1/2 onion, thinly sliced
- 1/2 cup snow peas
- 2 cups cooked brown rice
- 2 cloves garlic, minced
- 2 tablespoons soy sauce (low sodium recommended)
- 1 tablespoon vegetable oil
- 1 teaspoon ginger, minced Salt and pepper to taste

Cooking Time:

Approximately 20 minutes

Preparation:

1. In a large skillet or wok, heat the vegetable oil on medium-high.
2. Cook tofu cubes till golden brown on all sides, about 5-7 minutes. Remove the tofu from the skillet and put aside.
3. In the same skillet, combine the garlic and ginger. Sauté until aromatic, about 1 minute. Add the onions, bell peppers, and snow peas to the skillet. Stir-fry for 3-4 minutes, until the vegetables are soft and crisp.
4. Return the tofu to the skillet and add the soy sauce. Stir well to incorporate, then simmer for another 2 minutes.
5. Serve the stir-fried tofu and vegetables with cooked brown rice. Season with salt and pepper to taste.

Nutritional Value:
- Calories: Approximately 350 per serving
- Protein: Approximately 15g
- Carbohydrates: Approximately 40g
- Fat: Approximately 15g

6. Baked Cod with Roasted Brussels Sprouts and Wild Rice Pilaf

Ingredients:

- 4 cod fillets (about 6 ounces each)
- 1 pound Brussels sprouts, trimmed and halved
- cup wild rice
- cups water or vegetable broth
- 2 tablespoons olive oil
- Salt and pepper to taste Lemon wedges for serving

Preparation:

1. Preheat your oven to 400°F (200°C).
2. In a pot, heat the water or vegetable broth to a boil, then add the wild rice. Reduce the heat, cover, and simmer for 40-45 minutes, or until the rice is cooked and the liquid has been absorbed.
3. On a baking sheet, combine the Brussels sprouts with 1 tablespoon olive oil, salt, and pepper. Roast in a

preheated oven for 20-25 minutes, or until tender and gently browned.

4. While the Brussels sprouts roast, coat the cod fillets with the remaining olive oil and season with salt and pepper. Arrange them on a baking sheet lined with parchment paper.

5. Bake the cod in the preheated oven for 12-15 minutes, or until readily flaked with a fork.

6. Serve baked cod with roasted Brussels sprouts and wild rice pilaf, topped with lemon wedges.

Nutritional Value:

- This dish is high in protein from the cod fillets.
- Brussels sprouts are rich in fiber, vitamins C and K, and antioxidants.
- Wild rice adds complex carbohydrates and additional fiber to the meal.

Cooking Time:

Approximately 40-45 minutes for the wild rice pilaf and 20-25 minutes for the Brussels sprouts.

7. Quinoa Stuffed Bell Peppers with Black Beans, Corn, and Salsa

Ingredients:

- 4 large bell peppers
- cup quinoa
- cups water or vegetable broth
- 1 can (15 ounces) black beans, drained and rinsed
- 1 cup corn kernels (fresh, frozen, or canned)
- 1 cup salsa
- Salt and pepper to taste
- Optional toppings: shredded cheese, avocado, cilantro

Preparation:

1. Preheat your oven to 375°F (190°C).
2. In a pot, bring the water or vegetable broth to a boil before adding the quinoa. Reduce the heat, cover, and simmer for 15-20 minutes, or until the quinoa is cooked and the liquid has been absorbed.

3. While the quinoa cooks, prepare the bell peppers by removing the tops, seeds, and membranes.
4. In a large bowl, combine the cooked quinoa, black beans, corn, salsa, salt, and pepper.
5. Stuff each bell pepper with the quinoa mixture, compressing it tight.
6. Place the stuffed bell peppers in a baking dish, cover with foil, and bake for 25–30 minutes, or until soft.
7. If preferred, garnish the stuffed peppers with shredded cheese, avocado slices, and cilantro before serving.

Nutritional Value:

- This dish is high in protein and fiber from the quinoa and black beans.
- Bell peppers are rich in vitamins A and C, while corn adds additional fiber and nutrients. Salsa provides flavor without added fat or calories.

Cooking Time:
Approximately 15-20 minutes for cooking quinoa, and 25-30 minutes for baking the stuffed peppers.

8. Turkey and Vegetable Kebabs served with Couscous

Ingredients:

- 500g turkey breast, cubed
- 2 bell peppers, cut into chunks
- 1 red onion, cut into chunks
- 1 zucchini, sliced
- 1 tablespoon olive oil
- 1 teaspoon paprika
- 1 teaspoon cumin
- Salt and pepper to taste
- 200g couscous
- 300ml chicken broth or water Fresh parsley for garnish

Preparation:

1. In a mixing dish, combine cubed turkey, bell peppers, red onion, zucchini, olive oil, paprika, cumin, salt, and pepper. Mix well to get an even coating.
2. Thread the marinated turkey and vegetables on skewers.

3. Preheat the grill to medium-high heat. Grill the kebabs for 10-12 minutes, rotating regularly, until the turkey is fully cooked and the veggies are soft.

4. Meanwhile, prepare the couscous according to the package directions, adding chicken stock or water for flavor.

5. Serve the kebabs over couscous, topped with fresh parsley.

Nutritional Value:

- Turkey is a lean source of protein, rich in B vitamins and minerals like iron and zinc.

- Vegetables provide essential vitamins, minerals, and dietary fiber.

- Couscous offers carbohydrates for energy and is low in fat.

Cooking Time:

Approximately 20-25 minutes.

9. Eggplant Parmesan with a Side of Mixed Green Salad

Ingredients:

- 2 medium eggplants, sliced into rounds
- 2 cups breadcrumbs
- cup grated Parmesan cheese
- eggs, beaten
- 2 cups marinara sauce
- 2 cups mixed greens
- tablespoon balsamic vinegar
- tablespoons olive oil Salt and pepper to taste

Preparation:

1. Preheat oven to 375°F (190°C).
2. Dip eggplant slices in beaten eggs, then coat with breadcrumbs seasoned with Parmesan. Place the oiled eggplant slices on a baking sheet lined with parchment paper. Bake for 25–30 minutes, or until golden and crisp.
3. Heat marinara sauce in a skillet until warmed through.

4. Serve the eggplant slices covered with marinara sauce.

5. To prepare the salad, toss the mixed greens with balsamic vinegar, olive oil, salt, and pepper.

6. Nutritional Value:

7. Eggplant is low in calories and rich in fiber, antioxidants, and vitamins.

8. Parmesan cheese adds protein and calcium.

9. Mixed greens provide vitamins, minerals, and dietary fiber.

Cooking Time:

Approximately 35-40 minutes.

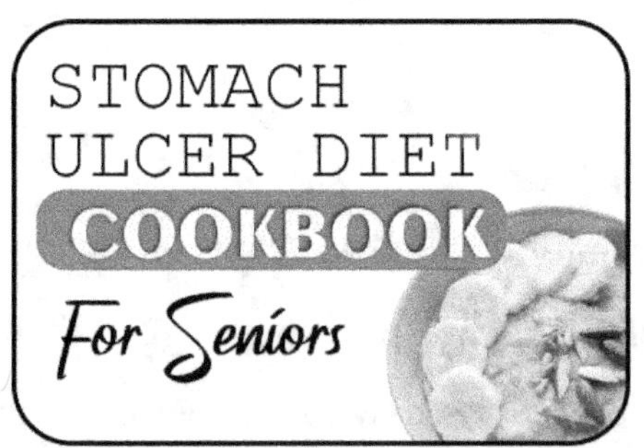

10. Lentil and Vegetable Curry served with Whole Wheat Naan Bread

Ingredients:

- cup dried lentils
- cups mixed vegetables (e.g., carrots, potatoes, peas)
- onion, diced
- cloves garlic, minced
- 1 tablespoon curry powder
- can (400ml) coconut milk
- cups vegetable broth
- Salt and pepper to taste 4 pieces whole wheat naan bread

Preparation:

1. Rinse the lentils and vegetables in cold water.
2. In a large pot, cook the diced onion and minced garlic until transparent.
3. Cook for a further minute after adding the curry powder.
4. Mix in the lentils, mixed veggies, coconut milk, and vegetable broth. Season with salt and pepper.

5. Bring to a boil, then reduce the heat and simmer for 20-25 minutes, or until the lentils and veggies are cooked.

6. Serve the dish with whole wheat naan bread.

7. Nutritional Value:

8. Lentils are a great source of plant-based protein, fiber, and essential nutrients.

9. Mixed vegetables add vitamins, minerals, and fiber.

10. Coconut milk provides healthy fats and flavor.

11. Whole wheat naan bread offers complex carbohydrates and fiber.

Cooking Time:

Approximately 30-35 minutes.

Here are 10 healthy snack recipes suitable for seniors with stomach ulcers:

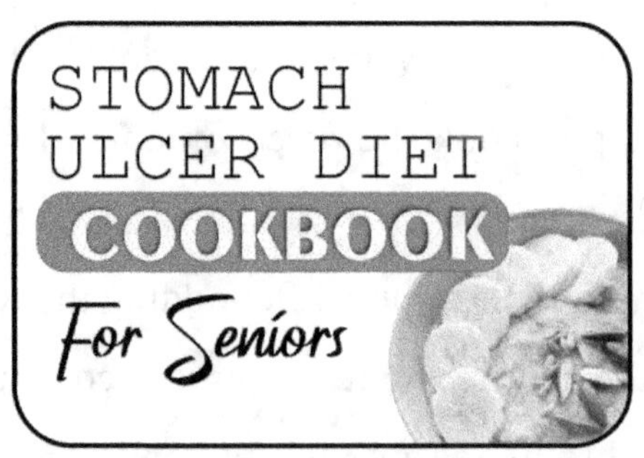

Chapter 6: Healthy snacks recipes

1. Banana and Almond Butter Toast:

Ingredients:

- 2 slices of whole grain bread
- 2 tablespoons almond butter
- 1 banana, sliced 1 teaspoon honey (optional)

Preparation:

1. Toast the whole-grain bread pieces till golden brown.
2. Spread 1 tablespoon almond butter equally over each slice of toast.
3. Place banana slices on top of the almond butter. Drizzle with honey if preferred.

Nutritional Value:
- Calories: Approximately 300 per serving
- Protein: Approximately 10g

- Fiber: Approximately 6g Healthy fats from almond butter

Cooking Time:

Preparation time: 5 minutes

2. Greek Yogurt Parfait

Ingredients:

- 1 cup Greek yogurt
- 1/2 cup granola
- 1/2 cup mixed berries (such as strawberries, blueberries, raspberries) 1 tablespoon honey (optional)

Preparation:

1. Layer Greek yogurt, granola, and mixed berries into a serving glass or dish.
2. Repeat the layering until all ingredients have been utilized.
3. Drizzle with honey if preferred.
4. Serve immediately, or chill until ready to eat.

Nutritional Value:

- Calories: Approximately 300 per serving
- Protein: Approximately 20g
- Calcium from Greek yogurt Fiber from granola and berries

Cooking Time:

Preparation time: 5 minutes

3. Vegetable Hummus Wraps

Ingredients:

- 4 whole wheat tortillas
- cup hummus
- cups mixed vegetables (such as bell peppers, cucumbers, carrots, spinach) 1/4 cup crumbled feta cheese (optional)

Preparation:

- Spread 1/4 cup of hummus evenly across each tortilla.
- Arrange the vegetables on top of the hummus.
- If preferred, sprinkle with crumbled feta.
- Roll up the tortillas tightly.
- If you prefer, cut it in half.
- Serve immediately or cover in foil to keep for later.

Nutritional Value:

- Calories: Approximately 250 per serving (without cheese)
- Protein: Approximately 10g
- Fiber: Approximately 8g Healthy fats from hummus

Cooking Time:
Preparation time: 10 minutes

4. Oatmeal with Berries:

Ingredients:

- 1/2 cup rolled oats
- 1 cup water or milk
- 1/4 cup mixed berries (strawberries, blueberries, raspberries)
- 1 tablespoon honey or maple syrup (optional)
- Pinch of salt

Preparation:

1. In a small saucepan, heat the water or milk until it boils.
2. Stir in the rolled oats and lower the heat to medium-low.
3. Cook for 5–7 minutes, stirring occasionally, until the oats are soft and have absorbed the majority of the liquid.
4. Remove from heat and let aside for a minute.
5. Transfer the oatmeal to a bowl and top with the mixed berries.
6. Drizzle with honey or maple syrup as desired. Serve hot, and enjoy!

Nutritional Value: Oatmeal with berries is rich in fiber, antioxidants, vitamins, and minerals. It provides a good balance of carbohydrates, protein, and healthy fats.
Cooking Time: 10-15 minutes

5. Rice Cake with Cottage Cheese

Ingredients:

- rice cake
- tablespoons cottage cheese
- 1 tablespoon sliced cucumber 1 tablespoon sliced tomato Salt and black pepper to taste

Preparation:

1. Spread the cottage cheese evenly on the rice cake.
2. Top with slices of cucumber and tomato.
3. Season with salt and black pepper to taste. Serve immediately.

Nutritional Value: This snack is low in calories and high in protein and calcium. It provides a good balance of carbohydrates, protein, and healthy fats.

Cooking Time: 5 minutes

6. Avocado and Tomato Rice Crackers

Ingredients:

- 2 rice crackers
- 1/2 avocado, sliced
- 1 small tomato, sliced
- 1 teaspoon lemon juice Salt and black pepper to taste

Preparation:

1. Put the rice crackers on a dish.
2. Top each rice cracker with pieces of avocado and tomato.
3. Drizzle lemon juice on the avocado and tomato slices.
4. Season with salt and black pepper to taste. Serve immediately.

7. Apple Slices with Peanut Butter:

Ingredients:

- medium apple
- tablespoons peanut butter

Preparation:

1. Wash the apple carefully before patting it dry.
2. Cut the apple into thin slices and remove the core and seeds.
3. Spread 2 tablespoons peanut butter equally on the apple slices. Place the apple slices on a platter and serve immediately.

Nutritional Value:

Apples are a good source of fiber and vitamin C.

Peanut butter provides protein and healthy fats.

8. Carrot Sticks with Hummus

Ingredients:

- 2 large carrots
- 1/4 cup hummus

Preparation:

- Wash and peel the carrots.
- Cut the carrots into sticks about 3 inches long.
- Put the hummus in a small bowl for dipping.
- Arrange the carrot sticks around the dish of hummus.

Nutritional Value:

- Carrots are rich in vitamin A and fiber.
- Hummus is a good source of plant-based protein and healthy fats.

These snacks are quick, easy to prepare, and provide a good balance of nutrients. Enjoy!

9. Hard-Boiled Eggs

Ingredients:

- 6 eggs
- Water (enough to cover the eggs) Ice (optional)

Preparation:

1. Place the eggs in a single layer in a saucepan and cover with cold water to about 1 inch over the eggs.
2. Bring the water to a boil over medium high heat.
3. When the water reaches a rolling boil, remove the saucepan from the heat, cover it with a lid, and set the eggs aside for 9-12 minutes, depending on the desired yolk consistency (9 minutes for soft-boiled, 12 minutes for fully hard-boiled). Prepare a dish of ice water while the eggs boil.
4. After the eggs have cooked for the proper amount of time, carefully remove them to a bowl of icy water with a slotted spoon.

5. Allow the eggs to chill in ice water for at least 5 minutes before peeling.

6. Peel the eggs and serve immediately, or refrigerate them for up to a week.

Nutritional Value (per egg):

- Calories: ~70
- Protein: ~6 grams
- Fat: ~5 grams
- Carbohydrates: ~0 grams

Cooking Time:

9-12 minutes

10. Chia Seed Pudding

Ingredients:

- 1/4 cup chia seeds
- cup milk (dairy or plant-based)
- 1-2 tablespoons sweetener (honey, maple syrup, agave nectar, etc.)

- 1/2 teaspoon vanilla extract (optional) Fresh fruit, nuts, or seeds for topping (optional)

Preparation:

1. In a mixing dish, add the chia seeds, milk, sweetener, and vanilla extract (if using).
2. Whisk the ingredients until thoroughly blended.
3. Cover the bowl and refrigerate for at least 2 hours or overnight, stirring occasionally to avoid clumping.
4. Once the chia pudding has attained the desired consistency (thick and creamy), give it one last stir.
5. Pour the pudding into bowls or jars and garnish with fresh fruit, nuts, or seeds, if preferred.

Nutritional Value (per serving):

Calories: ~150

Protein: ~5 grams

Fat: ~8 grams

Carbohydrates: ~15 grams

Cooking Time:

2 hours to overnight refrigeration time

Day 1:

- Breakfast: Oatmeal with sliced bananas and honey
- Lunch: Lentil soup with carrots, celery, and spinach
- Dinner: Baked salmon with steamed asparagus and quinoa
- Snack: Greek Yogurt Parfait

Day 2:

- Breakfast: Whole grain toast with almond butter and sliced strawberries
- Lunch: Tuna salad wrap with whole wheat tortilla, lettuce, and sliced avocado
- Dinner: Stir-fried tofu with broccoli, bell peppers, and snap peas served over brown rice
- Snack: Carrot Sticks with Hummus

Day 3:

Breakfast: Scrambled eggs with spinach and feta cheese

Lunch: Quinoa salad with roasted vegetables and feta cheese

Dinner: Grilled chicken breast with roasted sweet potatoes and sautéed kale

Snack: Apple Slices with Peanut Butter

Day 4:

- Breakfast: Greek yogurt with sliced peaches and a drizzle of maple syrup
- Lunch: Turkey and avocado sandwich on whole grain bread with a side of carrot sticks
- Dinner: Veggie stir-fry with tofu, bell peppers, onions, and snow peas over brown rice
- Snack: Banana and Almond Butter Toast

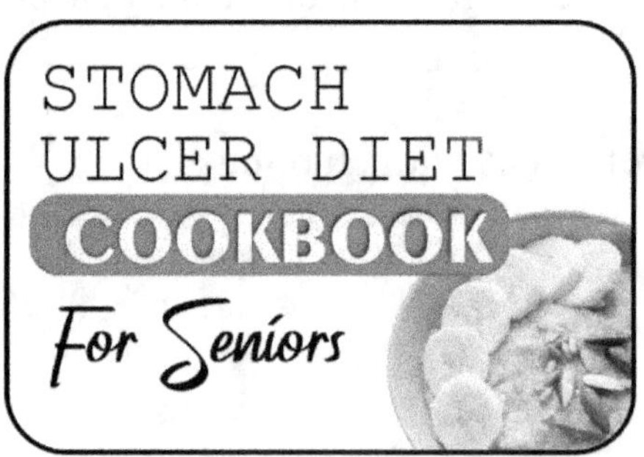

Day 5:

- Breakfast: Buckwheat pancakes topped with blueberries and Greek yogurt
- Lunch: Chickpea and vegetable stir-fry served over brown rice
- Dinner: Baked cod with roasted Brussels sprouts and wild rice pilaf
- Snack: Chia Seed Pudding

Day 6:

- Breakfast: Smoothie made with kale, pineapple, ginger, and coconut milk
- Lunch: Grilled chicken salad with mixed greens, cherry tomatoes, cucumbers, and balsamic vinaigrette
- Dinner: Turkey meatballs served over whole wheat spaghetti with marinara sauce
- Snack: Rice Cake with Cottage Cheese

Day 7:

- Breakfast: Cottage cheese with sliced avocado and cherry tomatoes on whole grain crackers
- Lunch: Lentil and vegetable curry served with whole wheat naan bread
- Dinner: Quinoa stuffed bell peppers with black beans, corn, and salsa
- Snack: Avocado and Tomato Rice Crackers

Day 8:

- Breakfast: Quinoa breakfast bowl with diced apples, cinnamon, and a sprinkle of chopped nuts
- Lunch: Salmon salad with mixed greens, strawberries, and a lemon vinaigrette
- Dinner: Turkey and vegetable kebabs served with couscous
- Snack: Hard-Boiled Eggs

Day 9:

- Breakfast: Poached eggs over whole grain English muffins with sautéed spinach and mushrooms
- Lunch: Whole grain pasta with roasted cherry tomatoes, garlic, and basil
- Dinner: Eggplant parmesan with a side of mixed green salad
- Snack: Vegetable Hummus Wraps

Day 10:

- Breakfast: Chia seed pudding with mixed berries and a dollop of Greek yogurt
- Lunch: Eggplant and hummus wrap with spinach, roasted red peppers, and cucumber slices
- Dinner: Stir-fried tofu with broccoli, bell peppers, and snap peas served over brown rice
- Snack: Oatmeal with Berries

Day 11:

- Breakfast: Oatmeal with sliced bananas and honey

- Lunch: Lentil soup with carrots, celery, and spinach

- Dinner: Baked salmon with steamed asparagus and quinoa

- Snack: Greek Yogurt Parfait

Day 12:

- Breakfast: Whole grain toast with almond butter and sliced strawberries

- Lunch: Tuna salad wrap with whole wheat tortilla, lettuce, and sliced avocado

- Dinner: Stir-fried tofu with broccoli, bell peppers, and snap peas served over brown rice

- Snack: Carrot Sticks with Hummus

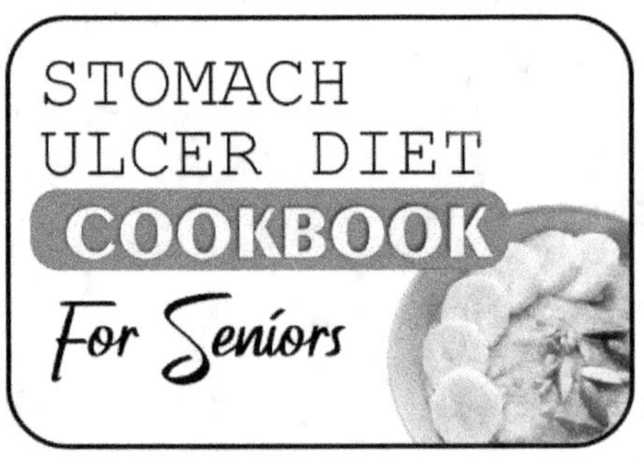

Day 13:

- Breakfast: Scrambled eggs with spinach and feta cheese
- Lunch: Quinoa salad with roasted vegetables and feta cheese
- Dinner: Grilled chicken breast with roasted sweet potatoes and sautéed kale
- Snack: Apple Slices with Peanut Butter

Day 14:

- Breakfast: Greek yogurt with sliced peaches and a drizzle of maple syrup
- Lunch: Turkey and avocado sandwich on whole grain bread with a side of carrot sticks
- Dinner: Veggie stir-fry with tofu, bell peppers, onions, and snow peas over brown rice
- Snack: Banana and Almond Butter Toast

Day 15:

- Breakfast: Buckwheat pancakes topped with blueberries and Greek yogurt
- Lunch: Chickpea and vegetable stir-fry served over brown rice
- Dinner: Baked cod with roasted Brussels sprouts and wild rice pilaf
- Snack: Chia Seed Pudding

Day 16:

- Breakfast: Smoothie made with kale, pineapple, ginger, and coconut milk
- Lunch: Grilled chicken salad with mixed greens, cherry tomatoes, cucumbers, and balsamic vinaigrette
- Dinner: Turkey meatballs served over whole wheat spaghetti with marinara sauce
- Snack: Rice Cake with Cottage Cheese

Day 17:

- Breakfast: Cottage cheese with sliced avocado and cherry tomatoes on whole grain crackers
- Lunch: Lentil and vegetable curry served with whole wheat naan bread
- Dinner: Quinoa stuffed bell peppers with black beans, corn, and salsa
- Snack: Avocado and Tomato Rice Crackers

Day 18:

- Breakfast: Quinoa breakfast bowl with diced apples, cinnamon, and a sprinkle of chopped nuts
- Lunch: Salmon salad with mixed greens, strawberries, and a lemon vinaigrette
- Dinner: Turkey and vegetable kebabs served with couscous
- Snack: Hard-Boiled Eggs

Day 19:

- Breakfast: Poached eggs over whole grain English muffins with sautéed spinach and mushrooms
- Lunch: Whole grain pasta with roasted cherry tomatoes, garlic, and basil
- Dinner: Eggplant parmesan with a side of mixed green salad
- Snack: Vegetable Hummus Wraps

Day 20:

- Breakfast: Chia seed pudding with mixed berries and a dollop of Greek yogurt
- Lunch: Eggplant and hummus wrap with spinach, roasted red peppers, and cucumber slices
- Dinner: Stir-fried tofu with broccoli, bell peppers, and snap peas served over brown rice
- Snack: Oatmeal with Berries

Day 21:

- Breakfast: Oatmeal with sliced bananas and honey
- Lunch: Lentil soup with carrots, celery, and spinach
- Dinner: Baked salmon with steamed asparagus and quinoa
- Snack: Greek Yogurt Parfait

Day 22:

- Breakfast: Whole grain toast with almond butter and sliced strawberries
- Lunch: Tuna salad wrap with whole wheat tortilla, lettuce, and sliced avocado
- Dinner: Stir-fried tofu with broccoli, bell peppers, and snap peas served over brown rice
- Snack: Carrot Sticks with Hummus

Day 23:

- Breakfast: Scrambled eggs with spinach and feta cheese
- Lunch: Quinoa salad with roasted vegetables and feta cheese
- Dinner: Grilled chicken breast with roasted sweet potatoes and sautéed kale
- Snack: Apple Slices with Peanut Butter

Day 24

- Breakfast: Greek yogurt with sliced peaches and a drizzle of maple syrup
- Lunch: Turkey and avocado sandwich on whole grain bread with a side of carrot sticks
- Dinner: Veggie stir-fry with tofu, bell peppers, onions, and snow peas over brown rice
- Snack: Banana and Almond Butter Toast

Day 25:

- Breakfast: Buckwheat pancakes topped with blueberries and Greek yogurt
- Lunch: Chickpea and vegetable stir-fry served over brown rice
- Dinner: Baked cod with roasted Brussels sprouts and wild rice pilaf
- Snack: Chia Seed Pudding

Day 26:

- Breakfast: Smoothie made with kale, pineapple, ginger, and coconut milk
- Lunch: Grilled chicken salad with mixed greens, cherry tomatoes, cucumbers, and balsamic vinaigrette
- Dinner: Turkey meatballs served over whole wheat spaghetti with marinara sauce
- Snack: Rice Cake with Cottage Cheese

Day 27:

- Breakfast: Cottage cheese with sliced avocado and cherry tomatoes on whole grain crackers
- Lunch: Lentil and vegetable curry served with whole wheat naan bread
- Dinner: Quinoa stuffed bell peppers with black beans, corn, and salsa
- Snack: Avocado and Tomato Rice Crackers

Day 28:

- Breakfast: Quinoa breakfast bowl with diced apples, cinnamon, and a sprinkle of chopped nuts
- Lunch: Salmon salad with mixed greens, strawberries, and a lemon vinaigrette
- Dinner: Turkey and vegetable kebabs served with couscous
- Snack: Hard-Boiled Eggs

Day 29:

- Breakfast: Poached eggs over whole grain English muffins with sautéed spinach and mushrooms
- Lunch: Whole grain pasta with roasted cherry tomatoes, garlic, and basil
- Dinner: Eggplant parmesan with a side of mixed green salad
- Snack: Vegetable Hummus Wraps

Day 30:

- Breakfast: Chia seed pudding with mixed berries and a dollop of Greek yogurt
- Lunch: Eggplant and hummus wrap with spinach, roasted red peppers, and cucumber slices
- Dinner: Stir-fried tofu with broccoli, bell peppers, and snap peas served over brown rice
- Snack: Oatmeal with Berries

BONUS: 14 weeks meal planner

The Paperback of This Version Has a Free 14 Weeks Meal Planner

MY WEEKLY MEAL PLANNER

Date

	Breakfast	Lunch	Dinner
MON			
TUE			
WED			
THU			
FRI			
SAT			
SUN			

SHOPPING LIST:

TO DO LIST

NOTES AND TIPS

Conclusion

In conclusion, "Stomach Ulcers Cookbook for Seniors" offers a comprehensive solution tailored to the specific dietary needs of older adults managing stomach ulcers. By providing carefully crafted recipes, nutritional guidance, and a focus on easily digestible meals, this cookbook empowers seniors to take control of their health and well-being. With a variety of delicious options, it ensures meals are both enjoyable and gentle on the stomach, reducing discomfort and promoting healing.

Through the management of symptoms and adherence to dietary recommendations, seniors can experience an improved quality of life, free from the worry of exacerbating their ulcers. Ultimately, this cookbook serves as a valuable resource, offering not just recipes, but also support and empowerment for seniors navigating the challenges of living with stomach ulcers.

MY WEEKLY MEAL PLANNER

Date

	Breakfast	Lunch	Dinner
MON			
TUE			
WED			
THU			
FRI			
SAT			
SUN			

SHOPPING LIST:

TO DO LIST

NOTES
AND TIPS

MY WEEKLY MEAL PLANNER

Date

	Breakfast	Lunch	Dinner
MON			
TUE			
WED			
THU			
FRI			
SAT			
SUN			

SHOPPING LIST:

To Do List

-
-
-
-

NOTES
AND TIPS

MY WEEKLY MEAL PLANNER

Date

	Breakfast	Lunch	Dinner
MON			
TUE			
WED			
THU			
FRI			
SAT			
SUN			

SHOPPING LIST:

TO DO LIST

●............................

●............................

●............................

●............................

NOTES
AND TIPS

MY WEEKLY MEAL PLANNER

Date

	Breakfast	Lunch	Dinner
MON			
TUE			
WED			
THU			
FRI			
SAT			
SUN			

SHOPPING LIST:

TO DO LIST

- ....
- ....
- ....
- ....

NOTES
AND TIPS

MY WEEKLY MEAL PLANNER

Date

	Breakfast	Lunch	Dinner
MON			
TUE			
WED			
THU			
FRI			
SAT			
SUN			

SHOPPING LIST:

TO DO LIST

NOTES
AND TIPS

MY WEEKLY MEAL PLANNER

Date

	Breakfast	Lunch	Dinner
MON			
TUE			
WED			
THU			
FRI			
SAT			
SUN			

SHOPPING LIST:

- ....
- ....
- ....
- ....

TO DO LIST

....
....
....
....

NOTES
AND TIPS

MY WEEKLY MEAL PLANNER

Date

	Breakfast	Lunch	Dinner
MON			
TUE			
WED			
THU			
FRI			
SAT			
SUN			

SHOPPING LIST:

To Do List

NOTES
AND TIPS

MY WEEKLY MEAL PLANNER

Date

	Breakfast	Lunch	Dinner
MON			
TUE			
WED			
THU			
FRI			
SAT			
SUN			

SHOPPING LIST:

To Do List

- ....
- ....
- ....
- ....

NOTES
AND TIPS

MY WEEKLY MEAL PLANNER

Date

	Breakfast	Lunch	Dinner
MON			
TUE			
WED			
THU			
FRI			
SAT			
SUN			

SHOPPING LIST:

To Do List

NOTES
AND TIPS

MY WEEKLY MEAL PLANNER

Date

	Breakfast	Lunch	Dinner
MON			
TUE			
WED			
THU			
FRI			
SAT			
SUN			

SHOPPING LIST:

●······························

●······························

●······························

●······························

TO DO LIST

································

································

································

································

NOTES
AND TIPS

MY WEEKLY MEAL PLANNER

Date

	Breakfast	Lunch	Dinner
MON			
TUE			
WED			
THU			
FRI			
SAT			
SUN			

SHOPPING LIST:

-
-
-
-

TO DO LIST

NOTES AND TIPS

MY WEEKLY MEAL PLANNER

Date

	Breakfast	Lunch	Dinner
MON			
TUE			
WED			
THU			
FRI			
SAT			
SUN			

SHOPPING LIST:

To Do List

NOTES AND TIPS

MY WEEKLY MEAL PLANNER

Date

	Breakfast	Lunch	Dinner
Mon			
Tue			
Wed			
Thu			
Fri			
Sat			
Sun			

SHOPPING LIST:

- ● -
- ● -
- ● -
- ● -

To Do List

- - - - - - - - - - - - - - - - - - -
- - - - - - - - - - - - - - - - - - -
- - - - - - - - - - - - - - - - - - -
- - - - - - - - - - - - - - - - - - -

Notes And Tips

MY WEEKLY MEAL PLANNER

Date

	Breakfast	Lunch	Dinner
MON			
TUE			
WED			
THU			
FRI			
SAT			
SUN			

SHOPPING LIST:

-
-
-
-

TO DO LIST

NOTES AND TIPS

MY WEEKLY MEAL PLANNER

Date

	Breakfast	Lunch	Dinner
MON			
TUE			
WED			
THU			
FRI			
SAT			
SUN			

SHOPPING LIST:

-
-
-
-

TO DO LIST

NOTES AND TIPS